# SOCIAL ANXIETY

## *How to Slay Social Anxiety*

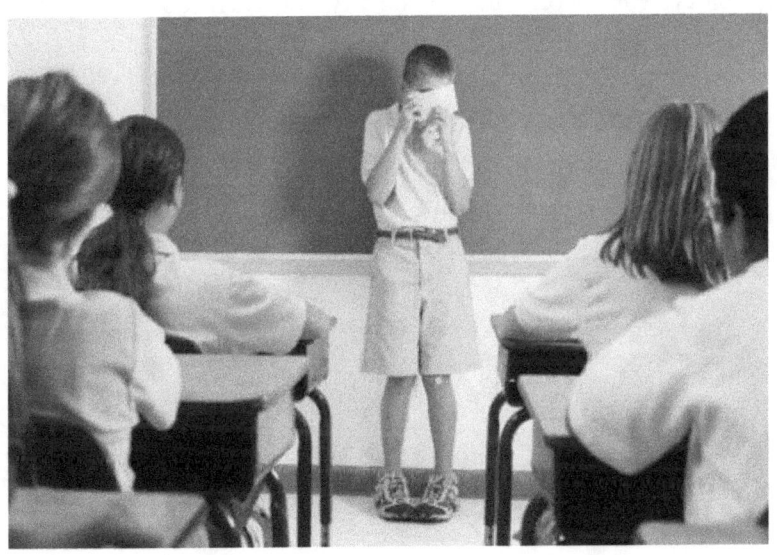

## By Patricia Carlisle

# Introduction

I want to thank you and congratulate you for choosing the book, *"SOCIAL ANXIETY: How to Slay Social Anxiety"*.

This book contains proven steps and strategies on how to slay anxiety disorder.

Mental health professionals had traditionally called severe social anxiety, social phobia. Recently the term social anxiety disorder has come into use.

We will use social anxiety disorder in this manual with one exception. We will describe how to overcome specific social fears like worrying that others will see your hand shaking while writing a check.

Because these fears tend to be much focused we continue to use specific social phobias to describe this aspect of social anxiety disorder.

Thanks again for choosing this book, I hope you enjoy it!

# TABLE OF CONTENT

# Chapter 1

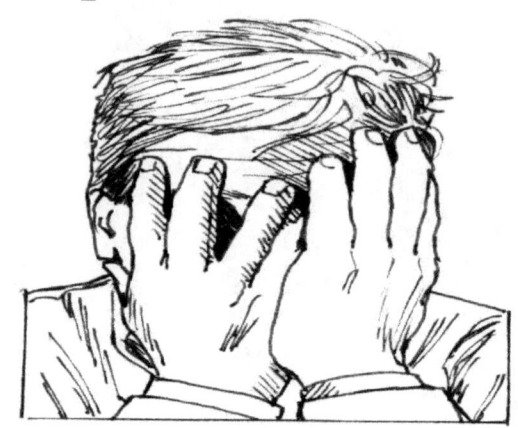

## SOCIAL ANXIETY

A definition of Social anxiety disorder was provided in 1994, by the American Psychiatric Association in the diagnostic and statistic manual of mental disorders.  Defines social anxiety disorder as a mock, and persistent fear of one or more social, or performance situations in which the person exposed to unfamiliar people, or possibly scrutiny by others.  The person fears that he or she will act in a way, or show anxiety symptoms that will be humiliating or embarrassing.  This mean that the heart  of the social anxiety disorder is anxiety due to concern about what other might think of you.

The social and performance situations feared by people with social anxiety disorder vary widely.  But the most command ones are public speaking, conversation with unfamiliar people, dating, and being assertive.

In addition, some individual with social anxiety disorder are afraid of eating,  or drinking in front of other people.  Being the center of attention, talking with supervisors, or other authority figures, urinating in a public bath room, usually only men have this fear, or intimate sexual relationships.

Regardless of the specific situation, people with social anxiety disorder share a common fear that others will think poorly of them.  Sometimes this worry about what others think is related to a fear of displaying a particular anxiety symptom such as blushing, or trembling. The following criteria must be met for an individual to be diagnose with social anxiety disorder.

1. The person must realize that the fear is excessive, and that most people will not be as frighten in a similar situation.

2. The person must avoid the situations that cause anxiety, or suffer through them despite great distress.

3. The social anxiety disorder must interfere with the person's life  in important ways, for example, keeping him or her from dating, going to school, doing well at work, or the person must me very upset about having the fears.

# Chapter 2

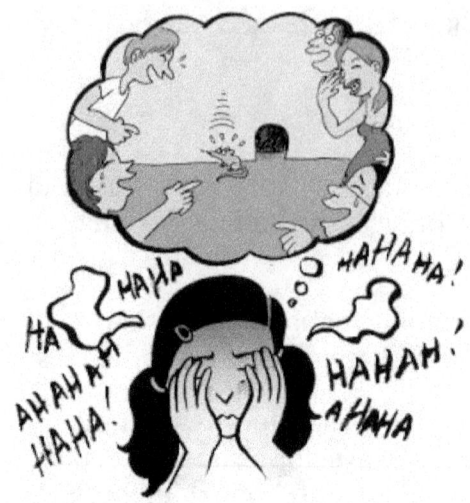

## INVEST IN CHANGE

No matter what anyone tells you making personal changes is hard.  And overcoming social anxiety is no exception.  To get as much out of this program as possible, you must invest both your time, and your emotional resources.

This means setting aside time at lease several times a week to work on your social anxiety, in addition to participating in a structured therapy sessions.  The work might include doing some of the exercises in this book, talking to someone you wouldn't normally talk with, or participating in the self help skills you will learn.  In fact, the more practice the better.  So if you can spend even 20 - 30 minutes a day you will see progress.

In addition to investing time, you must invest emotional resources.   By this we mean two things, first, some of the exercises in this book will make you feel uncomfortable, or possibly even very anxious.  Although it seems a little odd you must be willing to experience some anxiety in order to overcome it.

This means that you must face your fears in order to overcome them you do not have to face the worse one first, but you will have to gradually try some things you have been avoiding. Done systematically, that investment will pay off.

Second, you must invest emotionally by being honest with yourself, and with your therapist. As you start to analyze some of the thoughts and fears you have about yourself, and the world around you, you might find that some of them are embarrassing, or seem childish to you. Speak up about that, the thoughts and fears that cause you the most distress are the most important ones to talk about. Not talking about what concerns you makes your therapist job very difficult.

# Chapter 3

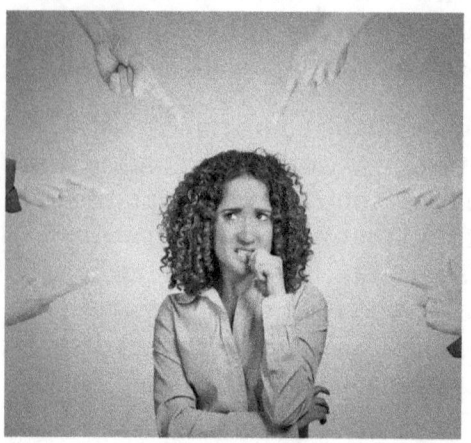

## PRACTICE AND EXERCISE

All of the exercise in this book has been carefully designed to help you progress through the program step by step. Most exercises build on previous ones, so it's important to do each one carefully. Once you have become an expert at all of the skills you might find short cuts that work for you. However, doing the procedures carefully first will assure that you have all the tools needed to cope with the anxiety you might experience as you try the more advance procedures.

The more you rehearse the exercises the more quickly the skills you learn will become new habits, and replace old problematic habits. And one of the best things about habits is that they require very little effort.

**PERSEVERANCE:** If you are like most people you have had problems with social anxiety for a long time, maybe even most of your life. If overcoming social anxiety were easy you would have done it already that is why it is important to stick to the program even if it does not seem to be working right away. We have included techniques to monitor your progress. Change usually start slowly, so pay attention to small improvements. Small improvements usually leads larger ones with time.

Patients, practice, and perseverance is the key. Be kind to yourself it is easy to focus on what you want to change, or things you don't do as well as you would like. It is not always easy to give yourself credit for your efforts. As you work through the program give yourself a pat on the back as often as possible. Look for things you're are making progress on, and celebrate them rather than betting yourself up for not yet reaching other goals.

Later we will devote a lot of attention to disqualifying the positive, because individual with social anxiety are often their own worst critic.

Most people find that being critical of themselves doesn't help them change it just makes them feel miserable.

**EXERCISE:** It's very important to know and understand how breathing can help with your mind, body, and soul. Breathing exercises are good for anxiety because it's fast, free, simple, and you can do them almost anywhere and at anytime. Here are three techniques that are commonly used for quick anxiety relief.

## Basic Breathing exercise:

1. Sit or stand in a relaxed position. Slowly inhale through your nose, counting to five in your head. Let the air out from your month, counting to eight in your head as it leaves your lungs. **Repeat**

## Belly Breath Exercise:

This is an exercise for learning to breathe abdominally comes from the University of Missouri, Kansas City Extension Center. Lie flat on your back to get the right sense of deep breathing. Place your hands, palms down, on your stomach, at the base of the rib cage. Make sure that the middle fingers of both hands are barely touching each other, and take a deep breath. Exhale, and begin again. For best result, practice this exercise for five minutes.

# Chapter 4

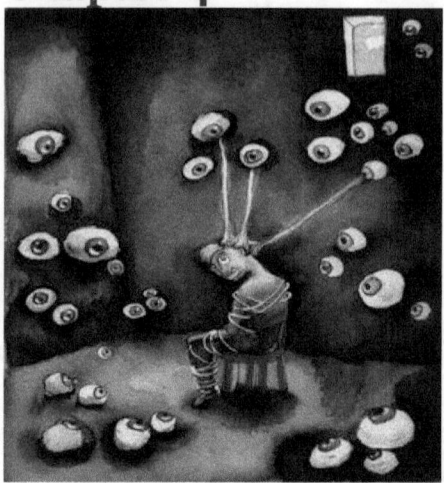

## FACING YOUR FEARS

One of the most helpful things you can do to overcome social anxiety disorder is to face the social situations you fear rather than avoid them. Avoidance keeps social anxiety disorder going.

### Avoidance leads to more problems.

Even thought avoiding nerve-wracking situations may help you feel better in the short term, it prevents you from becoming more comfortable and educated in social situations and learning how to cope. In fact, the more you avoid a feared social situation, the more frightening it becomes.

Avoidance may also prevent you from doing things you'd like to do or reaching certain goals. For example, a fear of speaking up may prevent you from sharing your ideas at work, standing out in the classroom, or making new friends.

### Challenging social anxiety

It may seem impossible to overcome a feared social situation; it can be done by taking it one small step at a time. The key is to start with a situation that you can handle and gradually work your way up to  more challenging situations, this will build your confidence and coping skills as you move up the "anxiety ladder."

# Chapter 5

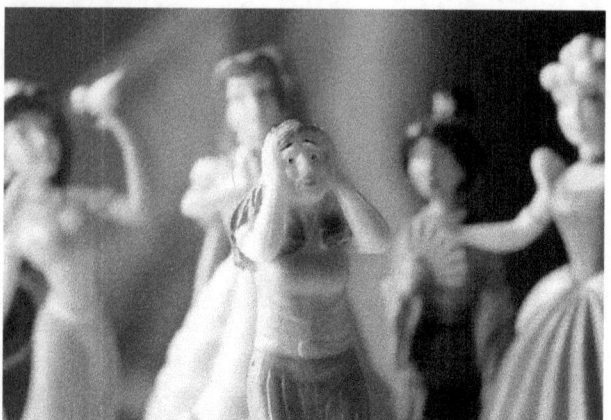

# BUILD BETTER RELATIONSHIPS

Staying busy is helpful for anxiety because it helps you to escape from all of your thoughts. When you're alone and quite, your thoughts seem to go through your mind, sometimes fast and sometimes slow. Anxiety has a way of controlling your thoughts weather they're negative or positive. Those individuals who have anxiety disorder tend to want to stay home and be alone. Sometimes just being around people can be a challenge. What you should be doing is creating good memories for positive thoughts.

It is important that you try to be around people even if it appears to be hard to do. If you do decide to be alone, try working on crossword puzzles, paint, make a phone call or draw a picture. The object is to try to stay busy and do things that will allow you to use your brain. When you're busy your mind learns how to cope with anxiety better. Try to avoid ways and places where you are alone with your thoughts.

Here are more activity tips to start you interacting with others in positive ways:

- Take a social skills class or an assertiveness training class. These classes are often offered at local adult education centers or community colleges. If you are not sure where to find them just ask your doctor or therapist

- Volunteer doing something you enjoy, such as giving food out at a shelter, teaching or tutoring, or working in a community store.

- Thing that will give you an activity to focus on while you are also engaging with a small number of like, minded people.

- Work on your communication skills. Good relationships depend on clear, emotionally, intelligent communication. If you find that you have trouble connecting to others, learning the basic skills of emotional intelligence can help. You can sign up for a communication class in community college.

# Chapter 6

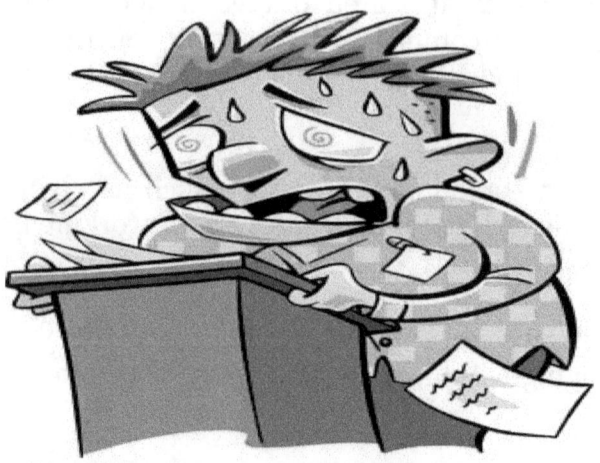

## IMPROVE LIFESTYLE BEHAVIORS AND HEALTH HABITS

Lifestyle changes alone aren't enough to overcome social phobia or social anxiety disorder; but they can support your overall treatment progress. The following lifestyle tips will help you reduce your overall anxiety levels and set the stage for successful treatment:

- **Avoid or limit caffeine.** Coffee, tea, caffeinated soda, energy drinks, and chocolate act as stimulants that increase anxiety symptoms.

- **Exercise.** You may need to change your exercise habits. Regular exercise, or no exercise, affects your overall heart health.

- **Drink only in moderation.** You may be tempted to drink before a party or other social situation in order to calm your nerves, but alcohol increases your risk of having a anxiety attack.

- **Keep a food journal.** When you write out what you ate for the day onto a permanent piece of paper, your mind takes a note of this and knows that it doesn't have to focus on food as much and eventually you'll stop thinking about the wrong foods and focus on the right foods to eat.

- **Quit smoking.** Besides being the leading preventable cause of death. Nicotine is a powerful stimulant. Smoking leads to higher, not lower, levels of anxiety.

- **Get adequate sleep.** When you're sleep deprived, you're more vulnerable to anxiety. Being well rested will help you stay calm in social situations.

Make sure all of your changes are something you can live with, and make small changes one step at a time.

# Conclusion

Thank you again for choosing this book!

I hope this book was able to help you to deal with social anxiety.

The next step is to try the coping skill and lifestyle changes.

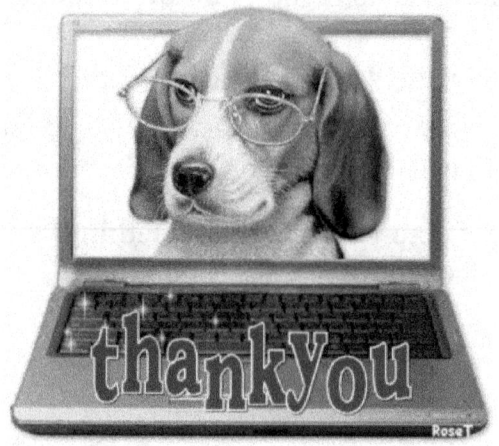

Finally, if you enjoyed this book would you be kind enough to share your thoughts and leave a review for this book on Amazon?

It'd be greatly appreciated!


Thank you and good luck!

# Preview Of 'ANXIETY ATTACKS:  YOU COULD BE A VICTIM'

## Chapter 1

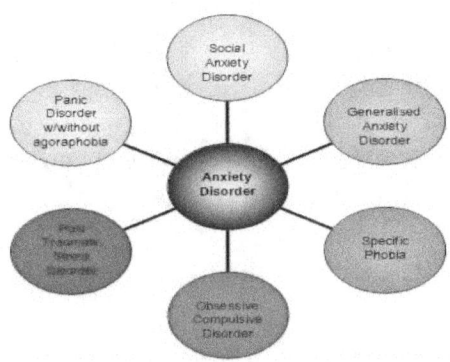

# CAUSES OF ANXIETY ATTACKS

An anxiety attack is a physiological reaction of the sympathetic nervous system, which creates the quick acting neurotransmitter adrenaline.  Adrenaline makes the signs of an anxiety attack, including fast heart rate, feeling bleary eyed and shortness of breath.  Reasons for anxiety attack are situated in mental and biological elements or factors that bring a person to this reaction

### PERSONALITY TRAITS

Being a perfectionist or vigilant creates a lot of physical and emotional strain.  These generally stable personality characteristics keep the sympathetic nervous system "on lookout."  This steady condition of activation expands the risk of an anxiety attack.

## COGNITIVE THINKING

Consistent and constant thinking of what could turn out badly or what was left untouched; being excessively worried about future objectives being met keep the sensory nervous system in a condition of arousal, expanding the danger for anxiety attack.

## DIATHESIS AND STRESSOR

Biological inclinations that increase the affectability of the sympathetic nervous system, the brain's piece that screens for threats, regularly are known as diathesis. It is a combination of this inclination and particular stressor that makes a person helpless or vulnerable that can increase the danger of a panic attack.

## INTENSE STRESS

The sound capacity of the sympathetic nervous system is setting up our body and brain in the time of danger. When we encounter intense stress that overpowers our capacities to cope, (for example, being injured), the reaction from the sympathetic nervous system may trigger a panic attack in a person, rather than sufficiently setting him up to confront the danger.

## ANTICIPATORY ANXIETY

Anticipatory anxiety is experienced by the individuals who have panic attacks all the time. This kind of anxiety is a worry of having an anxiety attack. The experience of having an attack is frightening to the point that the individuals who have them add to this continuous worry, which really builds the chances of having another attack.

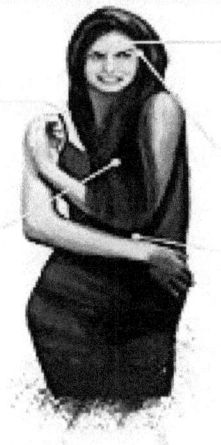

**ANXIETY ATTACKS**

SUDDEN, UNEXPLAINED
EPISODES OF FEAR

MENTAL
ANGUISH

DIZZINESS

HEART
PALPITATIONS

LOSS OF
APPETITE

**YOU COULD BE A
VICTIM**

By Patricia A Carlisle

To check out the rest of (ANXIETY ATTACKS:  YOU COULD BE A VICTIM) go to Amazon.com

# Check Out My Other Books

Below you'll find some of my other popular books that are popular on Amazon and Kindle as well. Alternatively, you can visit my author page on Amazon to see other work done by me.

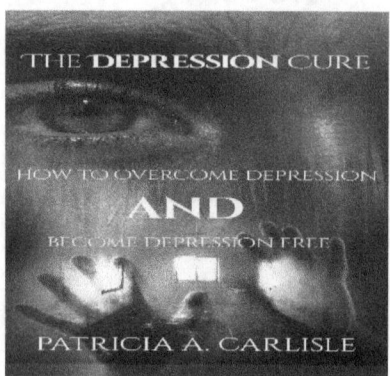

**THE DEPRESSION CURE: How to overcome depression and become depression free.**

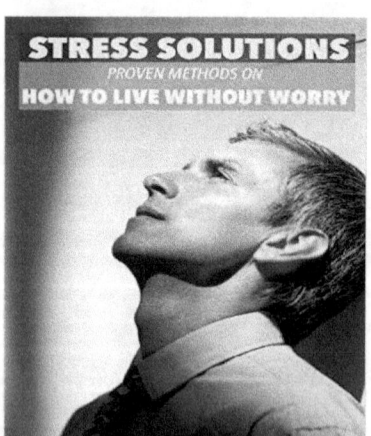

**STRESS SOLUTIONS: Proven methods on how to live without worry.**

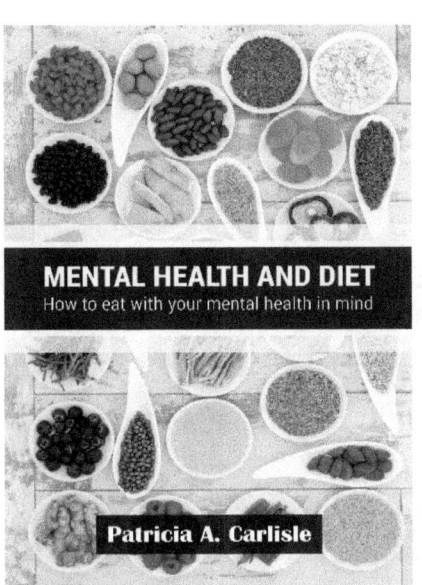

**Mental Health and diet: How to eat with your mental health in mind.**

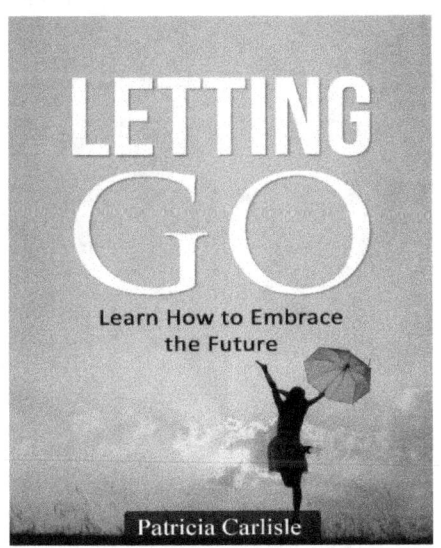

**LETTING GO: Learn How to Embrace the Future.**

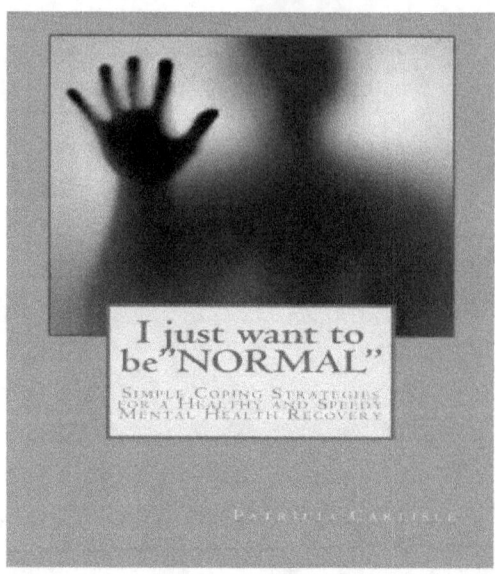

I just want to be "NORMAL" simple coping strategies for a healthier and speedy mental health recovery.

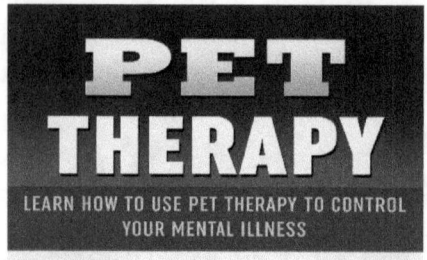
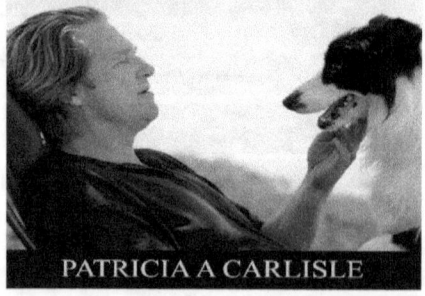

PET THERAPY: Learn how to use pet therapy to control your mental illness

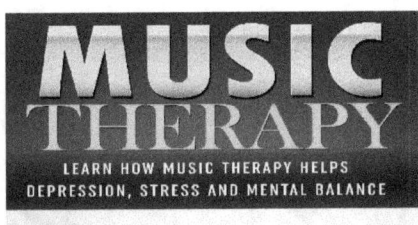

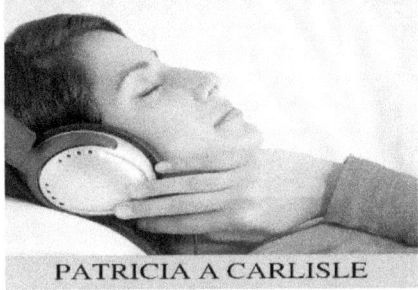

**MUSIC THERAPY: Learn how music therapy helps depression, stress and mental balance.**

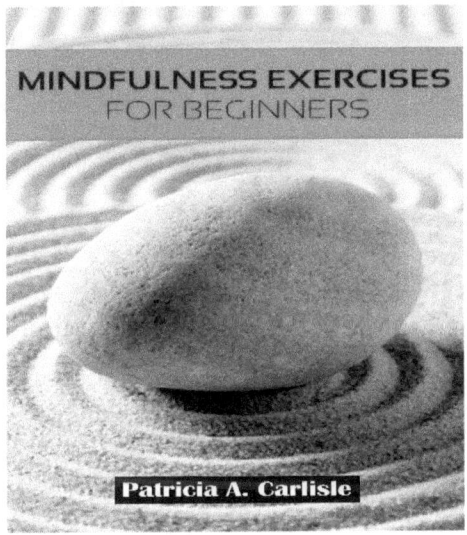

**MINDFULNESS EXERCISES FOR BEGINNERS.**

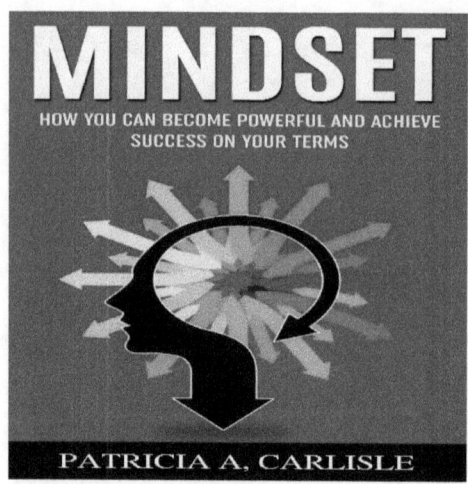

**MINDSET: How you can become powerful and achieve success on your terms.**

# BONUS: SUBSCRIBE TO THE FREE BOOK

## Beginners Guide to Yoga & Meditation

"Stressed out? Do You Feel Like The World Is Crashing Down Around You? Want To Take A Vacation That Will Relax Your Mind, Body And Spirit? Well this Easy To Read Step By Step

E-Book Makes It All Possible!"

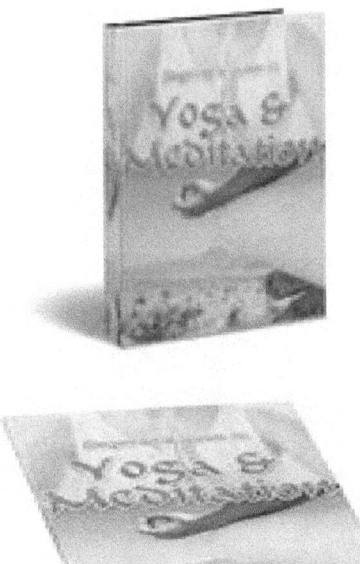

Instructions on how to join our mailing list, and receive a free copy of "Yoga and Meditation" can be found in any of my Kindle eBooks.

# NOTES

# NOTES

# NOTES

# NOTES

# NOTES

# NOTES

# NOTES

# NOTES

# NOTES

# NOTES

# NOTES

# NOTES